Living Fit Forever

"Creating *Your* own unique wellness lifestyle"

John-Eric Bonilla

ACE Certified Health Coach & Behavioral Change Specialist

John-Eric Bonilla

DEDICATION

This book is dedication to my wife Brita and my awesome kids Amanda, Stephanie, Arnold, Richard, and Isabella. The reason we want to live fit forever is to enjoy the time with those who make life so very sweet. Thank you my beautiful family for surrounding me with such incredible love; you are all proof that God is good.

CONTENTS

ACKNOWLEDGMENTS

Most importantly I want to honor the one and only Holy God and Savior Jesus Christ. Also my appreciation goes to those close friends who have inspired me to be better than I am: Julie Gross, who lives fit and lives a life of inspiring others and Rodney Ibanez, whom I met when I was 12 years old and who showed me by example what a good, selfless person of service truly is.

MESSAGE FROM THE AUTHOR

Dear Reader,

There have been many times in my own life that I have practiced unhealthy habits and behaviors that I mindfully did not want to do, sometimes for years. At other times I didn't practice behaviors that I earnestly desired to do. This wellness journey is about showing you how to modify your own behaviors and habits to match your desired outcomes—to live a fuller, happier, healthier, and more joyful life. It will not always be easy, but by the end of this journey, I am certain that all of you who truly desire to improve your state of wellness, health, and happiness will achieve incredible results in the quality of your lives.

As we go through this journey together up the magnificent mountain of wellness, I will be acting as your "sherpa," but it is your journey, not mine; I am just a humble guide trying to keep you safe, helping you make good choices, and keeping you continually progressing up the mountain. You will be making all the important decisions and choosing which paths are best for you to reach your ideal wellness lifestyle.

My final word of encouragement as we undertake this trip together is be strong and very courageous! You have the power and ability to change, to live a rich full life, filled with health, wellness and incredible joy. Do not settle for mediocrity. Embrace your destiny, and even more importantly, enjoy the journey!

Blessings always,

John-Eric Bonilla

WELLNESS PROPENSITY

What is a Propensity?

Merriam-Webster defines it as "an often intense natural inclination or preference."

Now the only issue we have here is what is a "natural inclination"? Is it something we are born with, or is it something that we learn? Does a baby have a natural inclination to nurse at his mother's breast before the breast is placed into his mouth and he experiences it? Does an alcoholic have a natural inclination for alcohol before he tastes that first sip of alcohol and the experience of euphoria that follows? Did you have a natural inclination for chocolate before you tasted and experience it? The answer definitely is no.

Most of our "natural inclinations" have a root cause or experience that lead us to practice that particular tendency, either to our betterment, such as eating vegetables and being active, or to our own self sabotage, such as watching too much television and eating excessive amounts of junk food.

If we don't currently possess the propensity to live our own wellness lifestyle, to be active, eat well, and live balanced by doing the actions that will make us flourish, don't worry we will develop them.

Now that we know that propensity is our *natural* inclinations, this brings us to our second question.

What is Wellness?

Let's talk with our old friend Merriam-Webster: "the quality or state of being in good health especially as an actively sought goal <lifestyles that promote wellness>."

Good Health

We should elaborate on two little words here, the words "good health." Should we take into consideration all aspects of good health? Good health is not just being able to bench press 200 pounds or being able to bend ourselves up like a pretzel in an advanced yoga class. Good health could be moving around free from pain, or maybe being able to chase our kids or grandkids around the park without coughing up a lung.

Not Healthy Lifestyles

As a child, I had a physical education teacher who was always running. Anytime of the day or night my family and I would be out driving in our small town, and we would see this guy running, running through town by the grocery store, running out in the valley miles from town, or even running in the pouring rain! He was a little high strung and ended up dying fairly young of a heart attack.

We all know the stories of world famous athletes who break all kinds of athletic records and are heroes to the world...until they are busted doping and abusing their bodies for performance results. Often we are crushed by the falling of our heroes. These are not healthy lifestyles or examples of how any of us should choose to live.

What is a Healthy Lifestyle?

This is a big question. I will limit our discussion to a few of what I consider to be the most result-oriented topics:

- Nutrition - what we put in our bodies
- Activities - how we move our bodies
- Mind/Body/Spirit – what we think, meditate, and dwell on
- Restore, Recovery, and Balance – how we rest, restore, and stay balanced

I Am Too Old to Change

We have all been told or said these excuses ourselves:

- I am too old to change to a healthy lifestyle.
- I like food too much to eat healthy.
- I don't have time to eat well and exercise, plus I can't afford it.

My Mom recently turned 76 years old. She retired about 16 years ago after working most of her adult life as a school teacher. She has always been overweight. When she retired at the age of 60, she was old. She used a walker to go places, and her appearance and countenance was of a tired old lady.

Fast forward to the present. Since Mom retired, she has been going to the gym every day except Sundays. She participates in the water aerobics class since it is easier on her joints. One day she proudly share with me, "This is day 4,000 that I have not missed a day at the gym!" For me the best part of this testimony is that she is no longer the tired old lady she was when she retired; she is vibrant and full of life with a sparkle in her eye and a joyful smile on her face. Let us learn from my mom—we are never too old.

The Purpose of This Book

At the time of this writing, I am a Certified Health Coach and Behavior Change Specialist with the American Council on Exercise, but this book is not to health coach you. I also hold a Certified Personal Trainer credential with the National Academy of Sports Medicine, but this book is not to train you either. In this book, I will not be coaching or training you.

My hope is that, through this book, you will achieve the ability to realize and implement your own root experiences and strategies that will promote your increased propensity for being well. By putting into practice these suggestions designed to improve your propensity for wellness in these four areas of your life, you will feel better, look better, be happier, and have more energy. You will also consistently experience more joy in your life.

At the very least, I will share with you what has worked for me. Over the last several years there have only been a handful of days each year that I did not feel joyful, thankful, and blessed. My days are simply amazing, and I wish the same blessings for you.

NUTRITION

When it comes to eating, there are some basic principles that we need to adhere to. At the same time, it is important to realize that there is no one-size-fits-all. Everyone has different preferences and requirements for their food. Some people are vegetarians and some vegans. Some people want to put weight on, and some want to lose a few pounds (sometimes a few 100). Many people have food allergies, and for some, certain foods that just don't agree with their bodies. So as you go through this chapter, remember to "make it your own." Eat foods that you love and that nourish your body and make you feel good.

The First Hurdle We Have to Make

There is a problem that most of us will encounter very soon after we start trying to eat better. That hidden problem is most of us, even though we don't know it, are addicted to food. If we eat wheat and white sugar as part of our regular diet, we probably have an addiction.

Let me give you an example. I went to stage two of eating 100% clean, deciding I would try if for five days, Monday through Friday. If I didn't like it

I would go back to my usual nutritional plan on Saturday. I felt so good after the first five days that I decided to extend 100% clean eating for a full 14 days. By the end of the 14 days, I felt 20 years younger; it was great. I then decided just to live this way for a while and see what happens. In week five on a Sunday, my wife wanted pasta. I made a delicious homemade red sauce with organic tomatoes, roasted garlic, onion, carrots, celery, fresh oregano, basil and parsley. But I did not want to eat the pasta and put white flour into my body. So instead, I lightly steamed some zucchini and broccoli and put the red sauce over it, and it was incredible. But my one big mistake was, as I was making pasta for my wife and kids, I bought them a big fresh French baguette. It looked so good I thought to myself, "One piece of bread with butter won't kill me." It did taste good, but when I woke up Monday morning I literally felt starving, and I was craving bread! During the four weeks before, I was eating so clean I never felt that hungry. Now after one piece of crusty French bread, I was starving. Now, do you think I was actually starving? Of course not; I was craving bread like an alcoholic craves liquor. After eating clean for the next eight hours, the craving went away. It made me realize that most of us have a food addiction, and we don't even know it. Most of us have eaten a big bowl of pasta, and even though we were full, we were still hungry for more. Addiction!

The good news is, once you break the bad habit of eating and living on junk food you will be free of a bondage you never realized you were in. In the words of Dr. Martin Luther King, you will be, "Free at last, Free at last!"

Foundation of life

This foundation of life is water. Our planet is covered by about 70% water, and our bodies are about 60% water as adults but a whopping 75% water as babies. Who do you think is healthier, babies or adults? We have all heard the saying, "Life grows where water flows." This is true. If we want to be as healthy, fit, and as full of life as possible, we need to drink lots of water to stay well hydrated.

A question we should ask ourselves is what is the leading cause of most diseases, sleeplessness, mental imbalances and aging? Our answer—dehydration. Water is the most crucial component in every type of cellular process in our bodies.

What is the recommended water consumption? I recommend you drink one full glass of water before going to bed and another glass of water when waking up. Also drink a full glass of water with every meal and snack. During the day we should be carrying water with us and drinking consistently for a total water consumption of about eight glasses per day. Even more is needed if we are exercising or if we live in hot, humid environments.

Is all water the same? Definitely not. We should always filter our water to help keep it and us as pure as possible.

Rocket Fuel for the Human Body

Imagine you have a beautiful sparkling red Ferrari parked outside your house. You go out open the door and slide into the seat. It hugs you sweeter than your mother ever did. You ignite the engine and it roars to life and then purrs like a jungle cat. You look down at the fuel gauge and notice it is nearing empty. Now my question to you is: Do you go and put in the cheapest gas you can find? Your answer to me should be, "No way, I want to put the best rocket fuel into my beautiful, high-performance vehicle that is available". This is exactly the attitude we should have toward- what we put into our bodies.

Now let's talk about your body. Most people say

they want incredible energy to keep up with a busy lifestyle and to do all the fun and exciting activities they desire to do. They say they want to look great, feel awesome, and wear clothing like a fitness model. Now the kicker is that most of these people say these things as they consume processed food products and live on fast food—from burgers and pizzas to cold breakfast cereal and highly processed nutrition bars.

Now picture you as a human Ferrari, a high performance person, with off-the-hook energy. You look spectacular and move like a sleek powerful jungle cat, graceful and strong. The first step to actually changing you into that human Ferrari is to start with the inside-out, which means feeding yourself "Rocket Fuel." I believe that even more important than your workout is what kind of fuel you are running on. Rocket Fuel for the human body is all natural foods, not modified but organic and pesticide free foods. If your food has a momma or grows out of the earth, it is probably good food. If it comes from a factory or has man-made ingredients you cannot pronounce, it is probably not good food.

The Very Best Foods

The very best things you can eat are

(1) Veggies

(2) Fruits

(3) Nuts & Seeds

(4) Clean Proteins

Veggies

When it comes to vegetables, fruits, nuts, and seeds, you want to eat a large variety with all the different colors of the rainbow. (Sorry, Skittles® don't count.)

To Go Organic or Not?

Let me put it plainly, GO ORGANIC!

The food and agriculture industries are the pushers of these addictive drugs, with their huge marketing budgets and vending machines selling sodas, chips, and candies everywhere we turn. Seventy to eighty percent of the average "American Western" diet consists of wheat, corn, rice, and soy the vast majority of which are GMOs (genetically modified organism) with sugar, salt, and chemical flavorings added. The majority of our beef, chicken, and pork are fed with GMO corn to fatten them up and increase the size and weight of the animals. All these unnatural processes serve to further contaminate our food supplies and decrease our health.

Do you want to put pesticides in your body? How about hormones and GMOs? I didn't think so. But with that said, it is needful to consider that organic is a lot more expensive, and many of us can't afford to buy everything organic.

There are compromises we can make to accommodate budget while keeping our overall health in mind. If we are purchasing produce that has thick skin that we are going to cut or peel off and throw away, much of the pesticides will come off with the skin. If we are on a limited budget and we had to purchase something for lunch, instead of an organic sandwich and organic potato chip, we could rather use the money to buy a non-organic salad with a non-organic chicken breast on it.

I have found that the more I eat organic and notice the difference in how it makes me feel, the easier it is to shell out the big bucks to buy it. But like everything else, we have to come to our own conclusions of what is best for us, we have to "own" our own wellness.

I'm No Kid

While serving as a trainer in one of the biggest gyms in Sacramento, I had a gentleman come and ask me about fitness. I mentioned the rocket fuel thing and about eating clean. I asked him, "Do you like vegetables?"

He answered, "No I hate vegetables," with a look of disgust on his face. He went on to say, "But I eat them because I am no kid."

I found this very amusing so I asked him a follow-up question, "What did you have for dinner last night?"

He answered, "Chicken and broccoli."

"Do you like broccoli?" I inquired.

The same familiar look of disgust crossed his visage as he retorted, "No, I hate broccoli."

I just had to follow up with one more inquiry, "Do you like avocados?"

He said, "Yes, I love avocados."

I then asked, "Do you like tomatoes?"

He said, "Yes, I love tomatoes."

Then I just had to inform him, "So you love tomatoes, and you love avocados, but you chose to eat broccoli which you hate."

I am sharing this story with you to go over our next very important point: food should be delicious! When you go to the grocery store or farmers market and you are looking at the produce, choose foods that look delicious. That is what you want to surround yourself with and have in your kitchen. If you eat just for health without taking into account your tastes and preferences, you are heading for disaster. You might set yourself up for a frustrating love-hate relationship with food. You can't rely on will-power alone as we all have a limited amount of will-power. Instead of running down your will-power reserves by eating things you don't like, you could be establishing healthy eating habits by eating healthy, delicious foods you enjoy and that satisfy you while making you feel fantastic.

Clean Proteins

When speaking of clean proteins, we will start with the best:

(1) fresh fish

(2) nuts, seeds, and Greek yogurt

(3) chicken and fowl

(4) beef, pork, lamb and any other natural hormone and chemical-free animal.

Clean protein is like the high-octane additive to the rocket fuel mixture. It provides us with more explosive energy. It increases the heat of your engine (body) to create a thermogenic effect resulting in a higher calorie burn. Proteins should be consumed at least three times each day, possibly more depending on personal lifestyle and exertion requirements (how much you move).

Milk and Dairy

If you are not lactose intolerant, and like me, you really enjoy a big glass of ice cold milk, you are probably asking yourself, "Is it rocket fuel or not?" Let us start with what exactly milk is designed for; it is designed to turn a 65 pound calf into a 400 pound cow in about a one year time frame. Some other facts about milk; Milk is a processed food, it does not come straight from a healthy cow to you, it goes through a lot of processing. Recent studies have shown that milk actually decreases the calcium in our bones. According to the "Save our bones campaign" and the "Physician for responsible medicine" we barley absorbs the calcium from milk and milk actually increases calcium loss from our bones and leads to an increase risk of osteoporosis. With that said milk definitively is not in our rocket fuel category, sorry milk lovers.

Since I went to 100% clean fuel, I chose to stop drinking milk. Like I said earlier, though, remember to "make it your own" by choosing for yourself what is good for you once you have all the facts. You will know what to do by how you feel. If you are not sure about a particular food item, cut it out of your diet for a week and see if you feel better.

Then add it back into your diet and evaluate how you feel. Trust yourself, and listen to your body. Often our bodies know better than our brains.

Fueling Times

I have heard many crazy stories from people trying to get in shape and lose weight. Things like, "I never eat after six o'clock at night," or "I don't eat at work." What most people don't realize is that if you go four or five hours without eating, there is a good chance that your body will think it is starving. When your body believes it is starving, it sends a signal to your brain saying, "I am starving!" Your brain then sends a signal back to your body saying, "Danger, danger we are starving! Let's hold onto our reserves of energy to increase the chances for our survival!" Now where does the body store its reserves of energy? That's right, in our body fat. Our fat is our body's energy reserve system. By not eating regularly, you just might be hindering your body's fat burning potential by slowing down your metabolism.

Just like you wouldn't drive a Ferrari around with ½ gallon of fuel in the tank, you don't want to drive your body around on near empty. The human body needs fuel (food) about every three to four hours. It does not have to be a lot; a few bites of some healthy, delicious food every three or four hours is sufficient.

The Crap Factor

We now know what rocket fuel for the human body is veggies, fruits, nuts, seeds and clean proteins. Most everything else is what we professionals in the health and wellness industry technically call "crap." If you are just starting to make the change from a normal diet of crap, I don't recommend going cold turkey. You might want to give yourself what I call "The Crap Factor." Picture everything you are going to eat today laid out on a dining room table. Ninety to ninety-five percent of what you see should be rocket fuel: veggies, fruit, fish, yogurt, lean meats, nuts, and seeds. The other five to ten percent can be anything you like—crap. This is your crap factor.

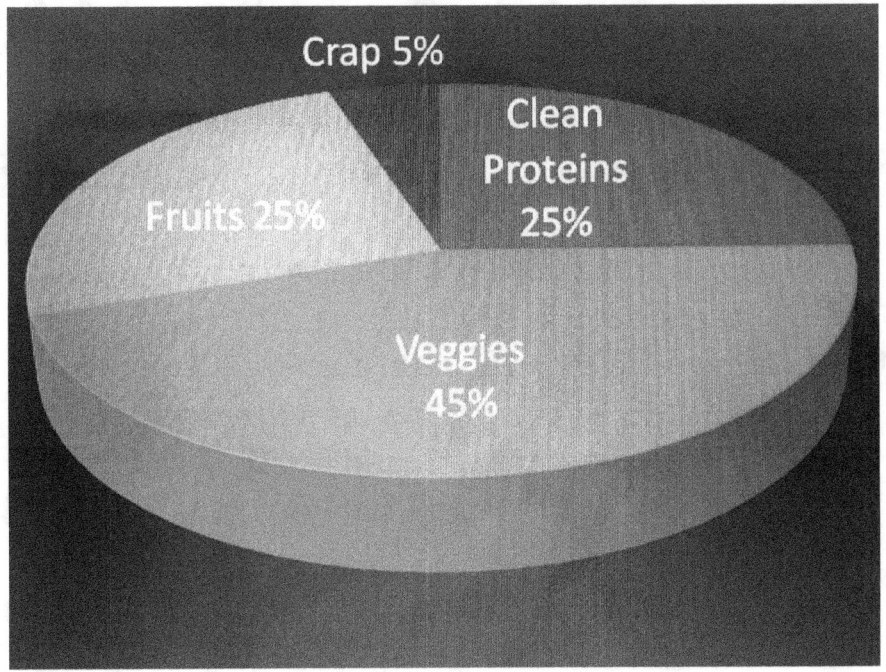

Do you want some bread (crap) in the morning? Go ahead. Do you want a piece of the birthday cake (crap) in the office for your coworker's birthday party? No worries. Do you want to swipe a piece of candy (crap) from your kids' Halloween bag? Sure, just don't let them catch you. Stay within the five to ten percent rule. Eat a little crap if you like; don't feel guilty. But as you do, tell yourself, "This is my crap for the day. Everything else is rocket fuel because I am becoming transformed into a high performance human Ferrari!"

Serving and Portion Sizes

Our standard serving sizes have grown over the past 50 years to crazy proportions.

Who really needs 32 ounces of soda or a 20-ounce steak? Let's talk about the appropriate portion size. With fruits, beans and legumes we want about ½ a cup. When it comes to starchy vegetables like potatoes and corn we should probably limit our portion size to about 1/2 cup which is about the size of a light-bulb, less if we are trying to lose weight,. And when we consider our super nutritional fuel (the bulk of what we consume) veggies and leafy greens we can generally go off the reservation and have as much as satisfies us, we just need to remember to have lots of different verities. A good measurement for nuts, seeds, and dried fruit is about ¼ cup, which will look like 2 golf balls. For meat, chicken and fish, an appropriate serving is about two to three ounces, which will appear about the size of a deck of playing cards. Depending on how much you move and your size, you might add an extra ounce or two. A large man of 6'3" requires more fuel than a petite woman of 5'5". These animal sources provide about seven grams of protein per ounce, so a three-ounce portion yields about 21 grams of protein.

Eating Propensity

The more you eat clean delicious foods, the more your body will get to like it. You will notice that your tastes will start to change, and you will start craving meals like a big, delicious, healthy salad with a nice piece of protein on top. My beautiful wife, Brita, makes an incredible chocolate cake. When we were first married, I would have one big piece and then go back for another—so delicious! Now when she makes it, and I take a small piece and have had enough after only a couple of bites. Heed my warning: as you eat cleaner, your propensity (natural leaning) will start going much more toward the clean healthy foods that make you feel so incredible, and you will not quite enjoy the crap as much as you used to. At this point, if you desire, you can bring your crap factor down to two to three percent or just one or two servings each week.

Once we have been eating like a Ferrari for somewhere between one week to twelve months, it is time to up our game!

Eating Phase 2: Super Clean

Our challenge, for this more advanced stage in our program, is to eat super clean—no crap at all—for five days, Monday through Friday. When we arrive to the weekend, we will have just a small bit of crap (one cheat meal). On the following Monday, the challenge intensifies to see how long we can go with total 100% clean eating. The more we do this, the more our body will like it. We will start to feel amazing, and the cheat meals will not be that attractive. Nothing will taste as good when compared to how great we will be feeling. At this point, we can have a cheat meal whenever we desire because we are clean-eating, highly-energized, vibrant human Ferraris.

Eating Phase 3: Intermittent Fasting

> ### !!!Warning !!!
> Phase 3 is NOT for pregnant women, those who are hypoglycemic, or those with any kind of eating disorder!

I know what you are thinking, "Didn't I tell you in the beginning of this chapter that if you go too long without eating that your body would think it is starving?" I did say that, but that is for normal people who live on crap. By this point, you should be well nourished and feeling great. If fasting is not for you, that is okay; just read this section and think about it. Remember also that I did say not everything I recommend is for everyone; you have to make it your own and discover what works for you.

Q: Why would anyone want to fast?

A: Because it has some incredible health benefits.

Some of the benefits of intermittent fasting include:

Normalizes insulin sensitivity

Boosts mitochondrial energy efficiency

Increases growth hormone production

Lowers inflammation

Lowers triglyceride levels

Helps shed fat and eliminates sugar cravings

Reduces oxidative stress

Increases longevity

Increases brain functions (BDNF and ketones)

Lowers blood pressure

Cleans and detoxifies the body so it can run more efficiently

During intermittent fasting, you don't want to restrict your daily calorie intake, you only want to restrict the time you eat. Some will fast 2-5, that is they will fast for two days and then eat normally for 5 days. Then there is 1-1 which is fasting one day and eating the next, alternating back and forth. Then there is 16-8 fasting, that's daily fasting for sixteen hours and eating for eight hours. These eight hours are our feeding window. This is the one **I recommend** because if you sleep for 8 hours you really only fast for about eight of your awake hours.

Start Slow

You should start slow, maybe try to make your eating window ten hours instead of eight. Once that gets easy, try reducing the window to nine hours. Once that is a breeze, you are ready for the eight hours. You can also try intermittent fasting on the weekends, and if you go outside of your feeding window, don't be too hard on yourself. Many people will intermittently fast during weekdays and then eat however they like on weekends. I believe getting started by fasting one day a couple times each month is fine. Once you start getting used to it, maybe extend your fast for a few days at a time.

Even if you just fast one day every month or two, you will still reap some health benefits.

RECIPES & FOOD

As we go through the recipes listed in *Appendix A* let's remember to make them our own, to be creative and use raw, healthy, natural ingredients that will help us thrive.

Fat

Everyone is scared of fat because we all think that fat makes us fat. It doesn't. Many fats are good for us and a great source of energy. When it comes to the foods we all eat, there are only three classifications, period. There are proteins, fats, and carbohydrates. We have already talked about proteins, so let's move on to fats and then later we will chat about the really scary calories, carbs.

Lots of different foods contain all three classifications. Avocados, for instance, contain proteins (about 3 grams per avocado), fat (about 23 grams per avocado), and carbohydrates (about 13 grams per avocado). But when it comes to the avocado, as well as many other plant based foods we eat, we should also consider the bigger picture—something called phytonutrients. What are phytonutrients we ask? They are the healing nutrients and natural chemical compounds found in many plant-based foods. Even though the avocado is loaded with fat (23 grams) it is a superfood. It has good fats that help feed our brains, ward off diseases, and keep us healthy, not to mention a ton of phytonutrients.

When we eat processed foods, even though they may have started with healthy natural ingredients, many of the Phytonutrients have been processed out. So you end up with what we call empty calories, which are calories devoid of the good nutritional content that keeps us strong, healthy, and without disease.

So don't be scared of fat, but be afraid—yes, be very afraid—of the dreaded complex carbohydrates!

Carbs

I don't think any of us want to go over a science lecture about the different sugar molecules found in carbs and their differences, instead why don't we just cut to the chase.

Carbs are not bad. SURPRISE!

The carbs we want to stay away from for our

health and longevity are the processed carbs such as bread, quick and/or instant anything, foods you buy in a box (like cereals) or in a bag (like chips), and other foods that have a long list of ingredients which we can't pronounce and don't know what they are even if we could pronounce them.

But we don't want to focus on what we shouldn't be eating; life is too short to be so negative. Instead, why don't we try to keep our focus on the delicious, healthy carbs we can and should be eating and enjoying as the vast majority of our intake. Here are some of my favorite phenomenal carbs that we can all search out and enjoy:

- Eat lots of fruits, especially berries like strawberries, blueberries, raspberries, loganberries, cherries and any other ending in (rries).
- Also enjoy leafy greens and veggies. We don't have to limit what we eat here. If we really want a nice full feeling in our tummies, we can eat as much as we want. Let the good times roll!
- We can add to our list beans, legumes, and healthy grains such as brown rice, oats, buckwheat and quinoa.

Pantry Raid

When it comes to preparing and eating good food, don't you think we should try to make it as easy as possible? If we come home tired after a long day and there on the kitchen counter is a big box of Kellogg's Fruit Loops® cereal or a package of Oreo® cookies, it will be very easy for us to pollute our bodies with them. We are all susceptible to "triggers." The main trigger to eating crap is to have it in sight when we are hungry. Likewise, the trigger to eating rocket-fuel is to have it in sight and easily accessible when we are hungry. We should all seek to organize our kitchens and pantries to have the rocket-fuel in sight and easily accessible and have the junk-food on the highest shelve in the back behind the largest box of oatmeal—or just throw it in the garbage. This is what we call a pantry raid—organizing our kitchens to make them *Living Fit Forever* user friendly.

Cook Once and Eat for a Week

Keeping nutritious and delicious food that is easy to eat will sometimes take a little bit of planning. I like to over-prepare when I cook. If I am making a delicious dinner, I like to make three times as much as we will eat and then package the excess in nice containers in the fridge to make three or four future meals . If I am making chicken, I will make three times what we will eat and then use the extra for making salads for the coming week. You can over-prepare your quantity of food for the next couple of days to make life simpler for the following days.

Breakfast Choices

Egg Breakfast

When it comes to eggs, we want to eat only organic and free-range eggs. Do we want egg whites only? No way, Jose! The egg yolk may have a bad reputation, but all the good things of the egg are in the yolk. For example the egg yolk will increase good cholesterol or high density lipoprotein (HDL), which helps to heal the body when we are under stress. The yolk also contains all the vitamins and minerals that are hiding in the egg. Furthermore, the yolk helps to support hormones and regulate the body's cortisol (stress hormone) production.

Please see recipes in Appendix A

This brings our path to the next step in our wellness journey, namely our activities—those dreaded, grueling, brutal workouts! Read on.

ACTIVITIES

The First Hurdle We Have To Jump

Most of us have a problem with our activity level—one of two common diseases called Chair-itis and ETS (excessive television syndrome). We tend to sit too much and watch way too much TV. You may be thinking, "But TV is just so good. The plots have gotten better, and the special effects are off the hook, not to mention the quality of the actors." We also think, "My chair is just so comfortable. I have spent years molding the cushions to the shape of my big butt." We might really love TV and enjoy a good sit, but these things do not compare to living our own authentic lives where we are the heroes writing our own stories according to our own personal values and our own visions of who we want to be and how we want to live.

Activities

Let's start with a few questions. Should I do cross training? Should I do yoga? Should I lift weights? Do I have to sweat? Is it going to hurt?

Now let me answer those questions for you…yes and no.

When it comes to activities, there are a few factors to keep in mind. The first and the most important question when starting out is what do we really enjoy doing?

Don't you think that activities should be fun? You're right; they should be.

Would you rather go work (out) or go and play (out)? The more enjoyable your activities are, the more you will do them instead of just thinking about doing them.

Activities Plus

I absolutely love lifting weights. I enjoy a sweat-drenching cardio workout. When I do yoga with its deep slow stretching, it takes all the kinks and tightness out of my muscles and makes me feel twenty years younger, supple, and relaxed. I did not always enjoy these routines. I started out slow, and the more I did them the more I had a propensity (natural leaning) toward them.

I also love taking walks with my lovely wife, chasing my kids around the park, and wrestling around and dancing with them.

The hard, sweat-drenching workout we do is for yourself and helps us to recapture our youth with every workout. But the other activities we do with the people whom we love are what we call "activities plus." We get to spend quality time with the people we hold most dear. This is the sweet part of life; this is where our quality of life is enhanced. And we should all try to schedule as many of these "plus" activities as we can.

Start your activity regime by doing fun things with those you love, the most important people in your life. Get the "plus" going on first. Spend some time with the significant people in your life. This could include walking, playing tennis, skating, skiing, swimming, or whatever else you enjoy. Then add in some on-your-own activities. Experiment with different formats of exercise. Do you like to dance? Then dance like no one is watching! Have you always wanted to try a boxing class? Then go and do it! Let your desire be your guide. Just jump in and start something—anything. Even if you discover you don't like it, you will have lived a little more with the added experience.

Start Slow

In my youth, I was very fit and active. At the age of thirty-something, I was not in quite the same condition. Unfortunately, I did not realize how unconditioned I was. I went to the gym, lifted weights like I used to, and a few days later I was in the hospital. Medical professionals call this the "Weekend Warrior Complex." It is a common thing for the 30-something group, especially men.

Now, as a certified personal trainer, I know that when we start our activities, we should start slowly and gently. Beginning with a 20- to 30-minute walk that really gets your blood pumping and makes you feel energized is a good start. Then when that starts getting easy, add some brisk "power walking" into your activities. When this also starts to get easy, you could add in a walk/run with a little bit of walking and a little bit of running.

Listen to your body while performing your activities, and let your body be your guide. Often our bodies know more and better then our brains. When we are in such a hurry to get results, it is easy to burn out and give up altogether in frustration. It is much more important to start slowly, build on your success, and develop success momentum. This leads to an active, healthy lifestyle and living fit forever.

If you are taking a class (I am a big fan of classes), rest whenever you need to. You don't have to keep up with anyone else. If you need to modify (make more doable) your exercise, modify away! The fitter you get, the more you will enjoy working out. Soon, instead of modifying down an exercise, you might want to modify up (make harder) the exercise.

Playify

Whenever we can, we should try and playify our activities. What's more fun, running by yourself or chasing after your kids or grandkids at the park? What's more motivating, walking 10,000 steps a day by yourself or being in a Fit-bit® challenge with your friends and family were the first one to 10,000 steps gets bragging rights? The fun factor is why activities challenges are so popular. It does not really matter if you win but that you get in your physical activities along with a lot of fun and camaraderie. We should all try to be creative and think of ways to "playify" our activities.

Developing Your Activity Propensities

I had the privilege of training a de-conditioned client in a short-term program. During our first session as she was going through a full body circuit of lifting weights, she looked very uncomfortable. With the look of a deer caught in the headlights, she told me very seriously, "I don't think training is for me." I was as encouraging as I could be, and we both noticed over the next several weeks that she started getting really good at working out. In the sixth week, we met on a Monday and she told me, "I woke up Saturday and really felt like I needed a good workout. That's not like me!" she said with surprise. Her propensity (natural leaning) for working out had started. It was AWESOME!

The lesson we can all learn from her is that even if something is not enjoyable at the start, with a little perseverance, you can develop a propensity (natural leaning) for all kinds of things. Let's try to create propensities for those activities that are good for us—the things that fulfill us and feed our inner soul and spirit—rather than activities that are destructive to us, sidetrack us from our values, and tarnish our inner essence.

Exercise Blueprint

Start Slow

If you are worried about being very unconditioned, please consult your doctor to make sure you are able to start a program without hurting yourself. Once you have been cleared to start your fitness training, a great way to start is with the most natural of motion, ambulating, which is just a fancy word for walking. A leisurely stroll around the mall or through the park is ideal. Once you feel comfortable with a stroll, push yourself a little bit with some brisk power walking, trying to break a sweat and make yourself breathe a little more forcefully.

A Little More

When you feel like you are ready to up your game, here are a few basic workouts that you can perform at home with little or no equipment.

Blueprint of a Workout

The Warm-up

This is how you typically want to start your workout. The purpose of the warm-up is to get your blood pumping to warm up the muscles and decrease the chance of sustaining injuries.

Initial Stretching

After the warm-up, we then want to take a little time to stretch our muscles, thus further decreasing the chance of injuries. For this stretching, we want to perform what is called "dynamic stretching." Dynamic stretching is performing stretching while in motion which enhances blood flow and gets the muscles and body ready to do some work.

The Work

Now that we have warmed up the body and completed our initial stretching, we are ready to do the "work" in our workout! This is the fun part or the hard part, depending on how you chose to look at it; I prefer fun. What we actually do depends on our goals, what we are trying to accomplish. Many people want to focus on losing weight, others on putting on some muscles, still others would like to work on increased performance in a particular sporting endeavor, and some have the goal of being all around more fit. I will outline a few workouts for different goals.

The Cool Down

After we have done the "work," we want to take a few moments to cool down and de-stress the body. This is our "cool down period." At this point, we will do a few static stretches, which is simply holding a stretching position for a number of seconds. We may also engage in some controlled breathing and/or meditation techniques.

Listen to Your Body

As you go through your exercise program, be very aware of what your body is telling you. We all have limitations and ways our bodies don't like to move or bend. As you start to move in ways that are unfamiliar to you, listen to how your body feels, and you will be able to realize and differentiate a beneficial workout pain from a bad "I-shouldn't-be-doing-this" pain.

Please see workouts in appendix B

MIND-BODY-SPIRIT

The Mind

At the age of twelve I absolutely loved martial arts movies. Bruce Lee was the star of the silver screen.; I remember seeing him in *Enter the Dragon*. My friends and I left the theater kicking at each other while yelling "HI-YA!" David Carradine was an actor who played the character Kwai Chang Caine in the hit television series *Kung-Fu*.

After that, I started taking karate lessons at the local dojo (karate school). I was not very good in the beginning, but I can still remember vividly when my first sensei spoke these words of wisdom to me: "It is the mind that makes the master." As the next ten years passed by, whenever I was out jogging I would say in my head and out loud, "It's the mind that makes the master." When there were nights that I couldn't sleep, I would get out of bed and stretch my body and meditate thinking over and over again, "It's the mind that makes the master."

At one dojo where I trained as a green belt, there was a gentleman there who was a black belt candidate. His name was Larry, and he was just one step away from achieving his black belt. He taught me a lot. And then suddenly I didn't see Larry anymore. I just kept training at any studio that would let me. I read all the martial arts books by the old masters and watched karate movies. The whole time I kept saying in my head, "It's the mind that makes the master." I eventually achieved the coveted black belt, and then the second degree black belt, and then the third. My instructor offered to sell one of his dojos, and I jumped at the chance. While operating this dojo, I achieved the fourth degree black belt, which is when you earn the title "Sah-bum-nim," which means "master instructor." I realized at that time the saying my first sensei had told me was true. If you say something out loud, believe it in your heart, and meditate on it night and day, you can create your future.

Since then, I have learned that the opposite also holds true: if you don't believe you will achieve something as a certainty, then you will not achieve it.

While operating and teaching at my martial arts studio, my old friend Larry came in one day and asked if he could train with me. I signed him up. He was still a black belt candidate, while I had went from a green belt to a master instructor. I was able to help him achieve his first degree black belt.

Since we know the power of our thoughts and our power to create, it is critical that we don't waste this potential by dwelling on things that are beneath us or not in our own best interests. Let me give you an example. Money, money, money. There is nothing wrong with money, but when that is your primary focus, you might just miss out on the things that you really love and those things that have true value to you. I wouldn't trade my health, my joy, my incredible children, or my beautiful wife for a billion dollars. Choose what you focus on very carefully, and make certain that whatever thoughts you keep in your mind are in line with your true values, goals, and priorities.

Spirit and Soul

There is an ancient Asian proverb that says, "You are your own worst enemy." Another proverb states, "If you can control your opponent, you have strength; but if you can control yourself, you have true power." My favorite proverb along this same vein is from the Book of books, the Holy Bible. In Proverbs 16:32 it says, "He who is slow to anger is better than the mighty and he who rules his spirit than he who takes a city."

We need to always remember our top priorities and values. It is important to focus our minds on these things in order to create our ideal joy-filled wellness lifestyles.

In the Bible it talks a lot about meditating on the Word of God. The Old Testament was originally written in the Hebrew language, and the word in Hebrew for meditate also means to mumble something over and over again in the same way that for years I would mumble under my breath, "It's the mind that makes the master."

Many people make a big mistake in that they choose the wrong sort of things to meditate and mumble about. Things like:

"I am always in so much pain"

"I will never be able to get out of debt"

"My grandparents were fat; my parents are fat, and I guess it's just the way I am too"

"No one will ever love me"

These are perfect examples of what not to dwell on. I like to meditate on and mumble things from the word of God because it feeds my spirit. Scriptures like these are meaningful to me:

Joshua 1-9 NKJV
"Have I not commanded you? Be Strong and of good courage; do not be afraid, nor be dismayed, for the Lord your God is with you wherever you go."

2 Timothy 1-7 NKJV
"For God has not given us a spirit of fear, but of power and love and of a sound mind."

Philippians 4-6 NKJV
"Be anxious for nothing, but in everything by prayer and supplication, with thanksgiving, let your request be made known to God; and the peace of God, which surpasses all understanding, will guard your hearts and minds through Christ Jesus."

Philippians 2-14&15 NKJV

"Do all things without complaining and disputing, that you may become blameless and harmless, children of God without fault in the midst of a crooked and perverse generation, among whom you shine as lights in the world."

Sorry, I don't mean to get preachy, but these meditations are just so good! I simply wanted to share them with you my friends.

Choosing what we meditate on is a wrestling match being fought in our minds constantly. We must always remember the proverb, "You are your own worst enemy," and choose our thoughts and meditations very carefully. We need to choose to dwell on the good, the beautiful, the noble, and be optimistic and brave while we create our ideal wellness lifestyle.

RESTORE, RECOVERY & BALANCE

Ebb and Flow

We all have what are called circadian rhythms. These are normal 24-hour patterns of how we live: when we sleep, when we eat, at what times of the day we have the most energy and brilliance, and at what time of the day we are sluggish and not at our best.

For example, some people are like me, morning people, we jump out of bed at 4:00am feeling like a million bucks. After our morning shower, we feel like we can conquer the world. Our brains are firing on all twelve cylinders. It is the best time of the day for us to study and learn new things. This is our best time to be creative, think outside-of-the-box, and to come up with innovative solutions to challenges. This is also our best time to work out, when we are at our peak. By noon, we may feel like we are operating on half the energy we had in the morning, and with every hour that goes by, we feel a little less energized.

Conversely, many other people are not morning people at all. They don't feel their best until noon, or maybe even 6:00pm. Some don't really feel energized until nine or ten o'clock at night—the night owls. There is no better or worse; we all need to embrace who we are and adjust our lives accordingly for our own optimal wellness time schedule.

Smell the Roses

Similar to our circadian rhythms, we might also have noticed that even though we have roughly the same schedule for eating, sleeping, and activities, we have an ebb and flow to our energy. One week we may be feeling stronger, faster and brighter than ever, and two weeks later we may just not be quite as vibrant. Then low and behold, two or three months later we are feeling even stronger, faster and brighter than our last peak.

We all have these rhythms that we live and go through. The important thing is not to fight them, as they are natural, but to try and enjoy the cycles and seasons of our lives. When we go through a period of feeling a little sluggish and tired, we should try to enjoy the down time—take naps, sit and watch the sunset, stop to smell the roses, or enjoy a leisurely game of cards with friends and family. Don't fight how you feel; embrace it. At other times when we are at our peak, we can challenge ourselves—push past our old limits, move faster than ever, lift heavier weights, learn new things, or perhaps dominate on the basketball, tennis, or racquetball courts, challenge kids half our age to see if they can keep up with us, or run that half or full marathon we have always wanted to try. Life is short, so we have to enjoy the high tides in life as well as the low ebbs in life.

Sleep

Most of us don't realize how important and critical our sleep is. If we are sleep deprived, it increases anxiety, slows down our metabolism, increases hunger, and robs us of our energy. Lack of sleep has a deteriorating nature on our brains. Many people may feel very anxious, and this keeps them awake. Lack of sleep causes them to be even more anxious, which leads to even poorer sleep. This vicious cycle can repeat itself endlessly robbing us of being as mentally sharp as we should be and as physically vibrant and powerful as we ought to be. If this is you, there a few things you can try.

Powering Down Routine

First, we can plan for sleep. If we want to start going to sleep around 10pm, at 7pm we can turn off our computers, televisions, tablets, and laptops. The blue light that emanates from these electronics causes a decrease in our melatonin level which hinders our healthy sound sleep. After we turn off the devises, we can do something that will relax us and put us in a sleeping mood. We can put on some beautiful, peaceful music or cuddle with our children or spouse. We can read a good book or spend some time just thinking about how blessed we are, the people we love, and the good things in our lives. We don't all have to do the same things as there is no one-size-fits-all. Try to create your own powering-down routines before bed so that you can sleep like a baby and wake ready to conquer the world.

Recovery

The harder our activities and exercise and the more stress we have, the more recovery we need. During our busy schedules, it is important to give ourselves time to recover. Our bodies need time to recover from the stresses we place on them. For my recovery time, I like to practice yoga. If you don't like yoga, you could just sit on the ground or lay in bed and take your time stretching your body in ways that feel good and therapeutic. Maybe relax in the hot-tub with a glass of wine or a good book, or receive a massage. We all need to manage our own recovery time and come back to a place of balance. What will you do?

Self-Myofascial Release

Another great option for recovery is "self-myofascial release," commonly called foam rolling. The foam roll comes in different sizes and shapes. The most common is 18 to 32 inches long and about 6 inches in diameter. The process starts with lying on the foam roll, placing the roll under a tight, sensitive, or sore muscle. Then roll the foam roll over the sore area while digging it in deeply. Once we have located the most sensitive spot on our body, we just hold it there and rest while taking slow, deep breaths. This is when the magic happens. There is an organ located were our muscles and tendons meet called the "Golgi tendon organ" or GTO. Once we find the knot in a muscle with the foam roller and hold it there for 20 to 30 seconds, the GTO is activated causing the knot to go back into alignment with the other muscle tissues. While performing this foam role technique, we might experience a little pain, but it will be well worth it for the relief we will experience afterwards.

Restore

Relationships are Restorative

We are social creatures. We are made to be in families and communities and to communicate with one another. You might have noticed that when you come home to a loving spouse who listens intently to you with a sympathetic heart and holds you with loving tenderness after a long hard day of challenges at work, all your stress melts away, and you feel restored.

The other day my son Richard turned 10 years old. Several times during that day, I was overcome by how sweet the last 10 years with him has been. I remember holding him as a little baby and cuddling him till he fell asleep. I remember dancing with him many times over the years, sometimes in our front-room in front of the TV watching Phineas and Ferb, sometimes at restaurants with live bands, and sometimes as we drove in the car. I also recall all the simple times at home with him sitting on my lap as we ate, watched TV, or read a book. I was overwhelmed with how sweet and wonderful life has been. I am looking forward to the next 10 years watching him grow into a young man. Richard has a little sister, Isabella. Every time I come home from work, she hears me coming up the stairs. She waits for me at the top of the stairs and leaps into my arms, which takes away any stress that I may have been carrying.

As I said, we are relational beings. The problem many of us have is we don't cherish the people who are closest to us until we don't have them in our lives anymore; then we miss them. If we could only slow down a little and enjoy the precious things in our lives instead of chasing after the shallow things such as money, possessions, and our own ego-boosting ventures. We need to value and work on our relationships, appreciating the people we have in our lives. As my dear Grandmother Carmen used to say, "The most important things we leave behind when we are gone are the threads of love that we weave into other people's lives while we are here."

We all need to take time to make sure the people we love most know just how much they mean to us and how much we value our time with them.

Own Your Own Restoration

Restoring ourselves is kind of like recovery but deeper. Instead of an hour massage, restoring one's self might be more like a week-long vacation with your family where you can enjoy life, play with your kids, and live stress free.

Or it might be going to the local homeless shelter and feeding the homeless on Thanksgiving; or a church mission's trip were you take care of orphans or dig a well in Africa; or possibly something as simple as escaping your busy work routine during your lunch break to walk to the local park and read a good book in the shade of a tree. I have coached many people who have implemented strategies this simple and totally achieved a lot more joy and peace in their lives. I personally find time in prayer to be extremely restorative.

Restoring yourself is very personal, and only you know what you need. Many people know what they require to restore themselves and yet put it off until it never gets done. They end up living stressed out lives that are devoid of the joy they so long for. Life is for the living. Feed your soul; recover who you are; embrace and live your dreams while you still can. No one on their deathbed ever says, "I should have worked more." They say things like, "I should have spent more time with my family," and "I should have gone to Hawaii with my wife," and "Why was I always in the office instead of pursuing my passions and truly living to my dreams?" Don't make these mistakes. Live well now. Search your heart. Take the risk to make the leap to follow your passions—just DO IT!

LIVING FIT FOREVER MIND-SETS

There are certain mind-sets that will lead us to an enhanced state of well-being and joy, and there are mind-sets that will detract and steal from us the joy and wellness we seek. Our first must-have-mind-set is thankfulness.

Thankfulness

This is a state of mind, and it is a choice. In almost everything that happens, we can choose to see the good and be thankful, or we can choose to see the negative and be ungrateful. Let me tell you a true story. Several years ago, I went through some financial hardships. In a very short timeframe, I went from earning a guaranteed $10,000 each month and driving a BMW 700 series, to earning $15 an hour and using public transportation to get to work. While taking the bus for the first time in my life, I looked online to see were the bus would pick me up to take me to a neighboring town for my job. As I was walking to the first bus stop, I had my iPod ear buds in with some beautiful music playing. I was saying to myself, "Thank you, God, that I have strong legs and good health so that I can enjoy walking on a nice, sunny day." Unfortunately, what I did not realize was even though I caught the bus at the right corner, I caught it on the wrong side of the street and ended up going in the wrong direction! I felt like such a country bumpkin. I called my employer, and he drove over and brought me into work.

The next day, I felt much more competent as I got on the bus going in the right direction. On this second trip, I was even more thankful that for the first time in my life, I had the privilege to participate in a form of transportation that many people use their whole lives.

These experiences opened doors for me that led me on a path to attaining a certified personal trainer designation, a health coach certification, and to attaining the best personal fitness in my life. Being thankful is a mind-set and leads us up to better places then we can imagine.

Forgiveness

Many of us think that forgiveness is something we give to others when, in actuality, it is a gift we give to ourselves. Somebody does us wrong, and instead of forgiving them, we hold a root of bitterness in our hearts feeling wounded at the injustice done to us. Does this indignation pay them back for their transgression? Are they being appropriately punished for their wrongdoing? No. In fact, they probably don't even know that we are holding on to our wound. The only person being harmed by not forgiving is ourselves!

As we forgive, we are claiming our own freedom. We might have legitimate reason to be angry and be justified in saying things like, "You don't know what my parents did to me, or how they treated me" or "My boyfriend was such a jerk. What he did to me was horrendous." This may all very well be true, but by not forgiving the offender in our hearts, we are continually giving them power over us to steal our happiness and our joy. By forgiving them, we are declaring with our forgiveness that we are "baggage free" and are not going to carry the added weight of someone's transgressions throughout our lives. When it comes to forgiveness, don't wait. Do it as soon as you can, and live free.

Hope and Faith

We all have hopes and dreams for the future. Some of us might want to lose that last 10 pounds; some may want to put on a little more muscle. Some may aspire to go on a Hawaiian vacation with family, while others may dream of starting a business or of having a baby to fulfill their aspirations of family. The one thing all these dreams have in common is that in order to realize them, we must have hope and practice faith daily.

I have a great hope deep inside of me that by writing this book and sharing with you how to live a wellness lifestyle, I will be able to change the world one person and one family at a time. There is a faith that possesses my whole being that people all over the world will live more joyful lives because of what is written herein and by what I do every day coaching people to wellness. I send this book out to you with my hope and faith along with blessings and prayers that it will benefit you, that you will embrace your dreams, that you will have hope and faith in what you truly desire, and that you will live the lives you so richly deserve.

WELLNESS OF THE SOUL

In this final chapter, I will share with you my own journey concerning the wellness of my soul, which is the secret of where my joy comes from.

My whole life I have sought after spiritual truths. I have read many books on Buddhist and Taoist philosophies. I read the whole bible through twice before I was twenty, parts of the Book of Mormon, and parts of the Koran. I have read about and practiced many different meditation techniques throughout my martial arts and yoga training. Many of these religions do have grains of spiritual truths in them, but they tend to miss the whole picture.

It was my own personal experiences that finally decided for me the truth, not what someone told me or what I read about. The experience that brought joy to my soul and abundance and purpose to my life was meeting face-to-face with the manifest presence of the Most High God.

I have to share with you that He is overwhelming, and I was totally undone. But the best part about knowing God is that He is a loving Father who genuinely loves all of us, His children.

So, I know without a doubt that my joy comes from the One and Only Creator of heaven and earth—God the Father, Jesus Christ His only begotten Son, and the Holy Spirit of Truth who lives in all of us.

He has spoken to me, and I have been in His healing, life-giving presence. You can to.

We have talked about nutrition and what we put into our bodies. The word of God tells us, "Not what goes into the mouth defiles a man; but what comes out of the mouth, this defiles a man." (Mathew 15-11 NKJV) Our words have power, and it is important that we guard our speech. If we live complaining and being negative, we will not achieve the wellness and joy we seek. We should, therefore, strive to speak our gratitude and love for those around us and for the great, loving, heavenly Father we all have.

We have also talked about activities and exercise. Now exercise does indeed profit us, the bible says, "a little." (1 Timothy 4-8 NKJV) But when we perform selfless acts of services and give of ourselves to others who cannot reciprocate that kindness, we are blessed by our heavenly Father. He says, "What you do to the least of your brothers you do to Me". (Mathew 25-40 NKJV)

When Jesus died on the cross, the veil in the temple of God was torn from top to bottom. (Mathew 15-38 NKJV) This signified that the way to God was now opened to all, and we do not have to go through anyone except Jesus to find Him or speak to Him.

The bible says, "And you will seek Me and find Me, when you search for Me with all your heart." (Jeremiah 29-13 NKJV) This privilege is available to all of us at any time.

If you do not believe me, or if you are conflicted in your heart because of what others may have told you throughout your life, I have a suggestion for you that will help you find the clarity that I have found.

First find a quite place where you will not be disturbed.

Second humble yourself by getting on your knees or laying face down on the floor.

Third, seek God with all your heart; cry out to Him in the name of Jesus, and He will reveal Himself to you. Don't hold back.

Fourth, share with Him your struggles, burdens, dreams, and desires. Open your heart to Him, and ask Him whatever you like.

And finally and most importantly, listen to Him! He will speak to you in a quiet whisper in your heart. You will know without a doubt that He is speaking to you and what He is saying to you. Often I have found that what He tells me, I will hear echoed in all kinds of other ways shortly thereafter, e.g. on the radio, through friends and family, on billboards, or just in normal conversation. It is amazing how the ruler of the universe uses the universe to speak to us.

Speaking of living fit *forever*—it is more true when we are in God and He is in us.

I'd like to leave you with a few parting words from God's Word, the Bible.

John 8:12

> Then Jesus spoke to them again, saying, "I am the light of the world. He who follows me shall not walk in darkness, but have the light of life".

And finally,

God is love!

ABOUT THE AUTHOR

John-Eric Bonilla, a.k.a. Coach Eric, lives in Sacramento, California, with his beautiful wife Brita, son Richard, and daughter Isabella.

He likes playing with his kids, watching other people get healthier and happier, and just savoring every moment of life. He has a passion for a fast, brutal game of racquetball and loves to cook and serve others.

Eric is an ACE Certified Health Coach, Behavioral Change Specialist, Orthopedic Exercise Specialist and Youth Fitness Specialist as well as a National Academy of Sports Medicine Certified Trainer and a Master Martial Arts Instructor.

Besides performing as a Health Coach and Trainer, Eric teaches "Introduction to the Culinary Arts" at a local elementary school and volunteers as a health and fitness coach to kids in his community.

Eric's company Fight-Fu Fitness performs health coaching, group fitness training, and personal training to individuals and corporate clients in the Sacramento area and around the world who seek to live their own unique wellness lifestyle. Eric is available for public speaking on topics of health, wellness, fitness, and living to our full potential. He can be reached through the website

www.LivingFitForever.com

APPENDIX A
RECIPES

Egg Breakfast #1
Eggs and Avocado
Ingredients:

Slice avocado in about ¼ inch slices, scoop out of the peal with a big spoon, arrange artfully on a plate, lightly season with salt, pepper, and a bit of cayenne pepper.

Heat a non-stick pan on medium heat. Add to the pan a teaspoon of coconut oil.
When the oil is melted and the pan is hot, crack open your eggs one at a time and gently release the eggs into the hot pan.

Watch eggs carefully not to overcook, when the bottom of the egg has firmed-up skillfully slide a spatula under the eggs (one at a time) and gently flip over. In about 30 seconds, the eggs are done. Use the spatula to remove eggs from pan and place them onto the avocado plate, lightly season with salt and pepper and enjoy!

*Variations of this dish can also be done with Tomatoes or any other of your favorite veggies.

Egg Breakfast #2

Ingredients:

2 eggs

½ teaspoon coconut oil

1 avocado

to taste

Salt, pepper & cayenne

The Awesome Omelet

Place a teaspoon of coconut oil in a non-stick pan and heat to medium.

While pan is warming up, add 2 organic range-free eggs to a medium size mixing bowl.

Chop a ¼ inch slice of onion, a small handful of organic cilantro, and ½ teaspoon of a jalapeño to a fine dice.
Add the chopped ingredients, 2 tablespoons of water, a pinch of salt and pepper to the egg bowl, and beat till fluffy with a wire-whisk.
Add the egg mixture to the medium-hot oiled pan.

While omelet is cooking, chop one organic tomato to a medium dice & lightly salt and pepper.

After about 1 to 1 ½ minutes of cooking, lift corner of omelet to check for doneness. When a light golden color appears flip in half carefully. After an additional 30 seconds of cooking, flip omelet over for 30 more seconds. Then carefully slide omelet out of pan unto a plate, cover with the seasoned tomatoes, and enjoy!

Ingredients:

2 eggs

½ teaspoon coconut oil

1 teaspoon fine diced onion

1 teaspoon fine diced cilantro

½ teaspoon fine diced jalapeno pepper

2 tablespoons water

To taste salt & pepper

Egg BF#3 The Fantastic Frittata

Place a teaspoon of coconut oil in a non-stick pan and heat to medium.

While pan is warming up, crack 2 organic range-free eggs into a medium size mixing bowl. Here is the fun and creative part of making a Frittata. You can add any healthy and delicious ingredients you have in the fridge, examples are: Leftover veggies, chicken, fish, meat, fresh herbs. Some of my favorites are:

Onions, garlic, ground beef, chicken, jalapeños, avocado, broccoli, mushrooms, cilantro, parsley, oregano, tomatoes, peppers, and the list is endless! Chop your ingredients to either a medium or large dice. Add chopped ingredients, 2 tablespoons of water, and salt and pepper to taste into the egg bowl and beat till fluffy with a wire-whisk Add egg mixture to the medium hot pan. While the Frittata is cooking chop one organic avocado or tomato to a medium dice & lightly salt and pepper. After about 1 to 1 ½ minutes of cooking lift corner of Frittata and if a lightly golden color appears flip carefully over for an additional 30 seconds. Slide Frittata out of pan unto a plate and cover with the seasoned avocado or tomatoes. Enjoy!

Outrageous Oatmeal Breakfast

Ingredients:

2 eggs

½ teaspoon coconut oil

Leftover:

veggies, chicken, fish, meat

fresh herbs

To taste salt & pepper

When it comes to oatmeal, the more natural the oatmeal the more nutrition you are giving your body. The more food is processed, the less nutrition it has and the quicker it raises your blood sugar. I suggest making your own oatmeal at home, and I recommend organic steel-cut or Scottish oats.

Make your oatmeal exciting!

Want exciting oatmeal? Want to make boring old porridge enjoyable? Yes! Once the oatmeal is cooked, it is a blank canvas just waiting for a culinary artist to make it spectacular.

Garnish a bowl of oatmeal with:

Fresh blueberries, Chopped walnuts, Fresh strawberries, Pumpkin seeds, **Honey, Cinnamon, Apples, Bananas, Cherries, Sliced almonds, Hazel nuts, Pistachios, Sesame seeds, Pomegranate seeds, Fresh ground Nutmeg, A drop of vanilla,** Gluten free granola. The list is endless!

Be creative; embrace your inner Michelangelo and challenge yourself to see how outrageous you can make your oatmeal!

Ingredients:

Organic steel-cut oats

A pinch of salt

Choice of:

Fresh fruit

Nuts and/or seeds

Yogurt Breakfast

When it comes to yogurt, all yogurts are not created equal. We usually want to have organic Greek yogurt. Greek yogurt is higher in protein and contains healthy living probiotic cultures that are great for your stomach and digestion. Always read the label of your yogurt to make sure that it is not loaded down with sugar and/or chemicals.

Preparing Yummy Yogurt

Similar to Awesome Oatmeal, Incredible Yogurt is a delicious blank canvas just waiting for you to make it spectacular. Have fun; do your own thing by adding your favorite toppings. Just remember, no M&Ms®, no cookie pieces, and definitely no marshmallows! Keep the toppings healthy and delicious.

Ingredients:

Organic steel-cut oats

A pinch of salt

Choice of:

Fresh fruit

Nuts and/or seeds

Main Meal Choices (Lunch and Dinner)

For our main meals, we want to nourish our bodies with nutrient-dense foods. Ideally we want a lot of delicious veggies, a little clean protein, a serving of fresh fruit, and always with every meal at least one full glass of water.

Salads

It is hard to go wrong with a salad—crisp leafy greens, juicy tomatoes, creamy avocados, crunchy sliced almond, nut and seeds, and refreshing cucumbers. Like I said, it is hard to go wrong with a salad—unless it is loaded down with junk. The junk we are talking about is things like premade salad dressings and cheeses that are filled with chemicals and artificial preservatives.

What we want in our salads are a myriad of different colored veggies. If there are vegetables you particularly don't like, don't eat them and don't buy them. We want to have a love affair with our food. We want our salad to be beautiful and exciting to us.

Here are a few of my favorite salad dressing recipes:
Healthy

Caesar Dressing

(Caesar Salad pictured is garnished with grass fed organic steak, avocado, grilled onions and shaved parmesano reggano cheese along with a dressing that has been painted on.)

Start with the 3 egg yolks and whisk in:
3 to 4 tablespoons of extra virgin olive oil
Three freshly chopped garlic cloves
2 anchovy filets finely diced
Juice from ½ lemon
1 tablespoon of shredded parmesano reggano cheese
Salt and pepper to taste

If you like your greens flavorful without being drenched in dressing, you might want to try painting the dressing onto the leaves.

Ingredients:

3

egg yolks

3 to 4 tablespoons extra virgin olive oil

3

garlic cloves

2

anchovy filets

1

Tablespoon parmesano reggano cheese

1

Teaspoon fresh lemon juice

The Healthy Ranch-like Dressing

Start with a cup of plain Greek yogurt and whisk in:

1 tablespoon of fresh finely chopped dill

Three cloves of garlic finely minced

Splash of apple cider vinegar

Salt and pepper to taste

Use as a dip for your favorite veggies or on your preferred salad and enjoy!

Ingredients:

1 cup plain Greek yogurt

1 tablespoon fresh chopped dill

3 cloves garlic

Splash apple cider vinegar

salt and pepper

Vegetable and Fruit Smoothies

Smoothies are a great way to get a lot of high-quality rocket fuel in an easy-to-digest refreshing drink. Making a smoothie could be as simple as throwing a carrot, celery stick, some spinach, romaine lettuce, and an orange or banana into a blender. Or it could be as complicated as what I do, my Rejuvenating Super Smoothie. If you would like to learn the secrets to this fountain of youth elixir, search YouTube for "Rejuvenating Super Smoothie," and you can see how I roll every morning. The important thing to remember when it comes to making smoothies is to make it your own. Put into your blender the healthy, delicious foods that you like and make you feel good. I am sure you will soon have your own personal favorite. Just make sure to use lots of organic veggies.

Rejuvenating Super Smoothie

Instructions:

Place all ingredients in a Vitamix® blender.
Blend and enjoy!

When it comes to vegetable and fruit smoothies, it is hard to go wrong. Have fun. Add your favorite healthy fruits and veggies (more veggies than fruits please) into your blender and go crazy. Experiment and come up with your own special blends.

Rejuvenating Powder Blend

Combine 1 teaspoon each of the following:
spirulina
matcha green tea
moringa
ashwagandha
chlorella
hemp protein
chia seeds

Ingredients:

1 organic orange

1 small lemon

2 organic celery sticks

2 organic carrots

1 leaf organic kale

1 handful organic mint leaves

1 pinch turmeric

5 organic strawberries

¼ cup acai berries

½ cup organic coconut water

Rejuvenate PB

The Minty Pineapple Refresher

* Dairy and gluten free
Provided courtesy of:
Alex Nella, RD, CDE

Instructions:

Add juice concentrate and tofu, then the spinach and mint to the blender and blend until smooth.
Add banana and pineapple chunks and blend completely.
Serves 4

Nutrition facts for 1 cup (8 oz)
Calories: 143
Fat: 1.5 grams
Sugar: 22 grams
Carbohydrate: 27 grams
Protein: 5 grams
Potassium: 385 milligrams

Ingredients:

8 oz silken tofu

12 oz frozen pineapple chunks

6 oz frozen pineapple juice concentrate

1 cup spinach

2 tablespoons fresh mint leaves

1 banana

The Mediterranean Mint Dream

(contains dairy products with lactose)
Provided courtesy of:
Alex Nella, RD, CDE

Instructions:

Add juice concentrate and yogurt, then the spinach and mint to the blender and blend until smooth.

Add banana and pineapple chunks and blend completely. Serves 4

Nutrition facts for 1 cup (8 oz):
Calories: 141
Fat: 0 grams
Sugar: 23 grams
Carbohydrate: 28 grams
Protein: 6 grams
Potassium: 275 milligrams

Ingredients:

8 oz plain Greek yogurt

12 oz frozen pineapple chunks

6 oz frozen pineapple juice concentrate

1 cup spinach

2 tablespoons fresh mint leaves

1 banana

APPENDIX B
WORKOUTS

Basic Workout #1

Warm-up—choice of:

A brisk 5 minutes of running in place
Walking briskly outside for 5 minutes

Dynamic Stretching:

Walking High Knees
With each step, hold your shin just under the knee and gently pull it toward your shoulder. As you walk, alternate legs pulling the knee toward your shoulder.

Stretch Kick
Lightly and gently swing one leg up in front of you, keeping it as straight as you can in order to stretch your hamstring. As you walk forward, alternate legs.

The Monster Lunge
Take a huge monster step forward, placing your hand on your front thigh and sinking as low as you can, stretching through your hips.

All these stretches should feel good; don't overdo it. Start gently, respecting your body's limitations.

The Work

(required equipment—one stout kitchen chair or bench)

Chair Sit Downs

Place the chair behind you.

Sit back onto the chair, lightly touching your butt to the chair, and then stand back up with a nice tall posture. Repeat this action 20 times. Beginning this movement in the chair will help develop a good squat technique.

Abdominal Crunches

Lay on your back with your knees up and your feet flat on the ground.

Place your fingertips behind your head to support your neck.

Lift your shoulder blades straight off the ground. Keep your neck long by maintaining space between your chin and chest. Make certain not to yank on your head. As you lift your shoulder blades up, pull your bellybutton in, squeezing your abdominal muscles. Repeat this 20 to 50 times.

Stepping Back Lunges

Start with feet hip width apart.
Step back with one foot while placing your hand on your front thigh.
Bring back foot back to starting position. Then repeat with opposite foot.
Alternating legs, repeat this for about 20 repetitions.

Knee Push-ups

Lay flat on your stomach, placing your hands palms down under your shoulders.
Push yourself up onto your hands and knees and then lower yourself back to the ground. Repeat between 10 and 20 repetitions.

The Cool Down

Softly bend your knees. Take a deep breath, and as you exhale, hang down toward your feet and just hang a rest for about 30 seconds.
Roll your back up slowly, one vertebra at a time. When you arrive to a full stand, perform a big shoulder roll, rolling your shoulders back in a big relaxed motion.
Reach your fingers and hands up to the sky and just perform a big stretch, like when you wake up, arch back slightly, pushing your elbows together behind

your back.

From there lightly shake your body arms and legs releasing all your tension.

Basic work-out complete!

The Four-Day-Per-Week Strength and Muscle Building Workout

This is one of my favorite routines. For this workout, we divide the body up so that every major muscle group gets worked twice each week and gets to rest for the other five days to achieve increased strength and muscle development.

Repetitions and Weight

Questions:
How heavy should I lift, and how many repetitions should I do?

Answer:
It depends on your goals. If you want to sculpt and tone your body such as a fitness model, you would use moderate weight and high repetitions, such as 65%-75% of your one rep max with repetitions between 15 and 30 per set. Conversely, if you want

to really put on thick muscles, you would go heavy with your weights, such as 75%-95% of your 1 rep max, and your repetitions would be between 6 and 12.

Warm-up

Begin every workout with five minutes of cardio, whatever type you like. Some cardio options are:
Treadmill
Elliptical
Jumping Rope
Running
Core exercises
Stretching

Before every workout, also include one or more of the following:
High Knees
Stretch Kick
Spiderman Crawls
Lateral Walks

10 Minutes of Core Work
Do one minute of each of these core exercises:
Crunches
Twisting Crunches (1 min each side)
Tabletop Crunches
Flutter Kicks

Leg Lift
Scoops
Side Plank (1 min each side)
Prone Plank

The Work Monday and Thursday

- Legs-Chest and Triceps

- Dumbbell Squats

- Body Weight Lunge

- Chest Press

- Chair Dips

- Skull-Crushers

The Work Tuesday and Friday

- Back-Shoulders-Biceps

- Lat Pull-Downs

- Bent-Over Rows

- Bicep Curls

- Rotating Deltoid Press

- Front Deltoid Raises

- Lateral Deltoid Raises

- Rear Deltoid Raises

The Cool Down – After Every Work Out

Softly bend your knees, take a deep breath and as you exhale hang down toward your feet and just hang a rest for about 30 seconds.

Roll your back up slowly, one vertebra at a time. When you arrive to a full stand, perform a big shoulder roll, rolling your shoulders back in a big relaxed motion.

Reach your fingers and hands up to the sky and just perform a big stretch, like when you wake up, arch back slightly, pushing your elbows together behind your back.

From there lightly shake your body, arms and legs releasing all your tension.

Basic work-out complete!

Demonstrations of most of the listed workouts and exercises can be found for FREE at LivingFitForever.com

www.ingramcontent.com/pod-product-compliance
Lightning Source LLC
Chambersburg PA
CBHW071214280526
45787CB00002B/679

* 9 7 8 1 5 3 4 7 7 4 3 1 5 *